Live in Wellness Now
A Proactive Guide to Living Well

Be Present | Be Purposeful | Be Well

By **Barbara B. Appelbaum**

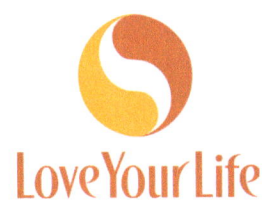

Live in Wellness Now Copyright © 2013 by Barbara B. Appelbaum. All rights reserved. No part of this book may be used or reproduced in any manner whatsoever without written permission from the author, except by a reviewer who may quote brief passages for review purposes.

For more information about this book or the author, visit:
http://appelbaumwellness.com/

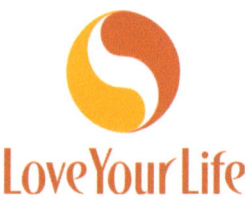

Love Your Life Publishing
www.loveyourlifepublishing.com

ISBN: 978-1-934509-70-8

Library of Congress Control Number: 2013930037

Printed in the United States of America

First Printing 2013

Cover design: www.Cyanotype.ca

Editing: Gwen Hoffnagle

Notice:
The information in this book is not intended or implied to be a substitute for professional medical advice, diagnosis or treatment. You are encouraged to confirm any information obtained from or through this book and review all information regarding any medical condition or treatment with your physician and members of your health care team.

Advance Praise for Live in Wellness Now

What a gift Barbara has created for all of us! Live in Wellness Now *finally puts forth a simple, no nonsense way for EVERYONE to focus on the single most important aspect of our lives, namely our health. In today's world, who among us can honestly say they understand their personal path to wellness? Behavioral change is the single most difficult thing for us to accomplish. While everyone is always looking for the "quick fix" in addressing their health,* Live in Wellness Now *FINALLY gives all of us a realistic roadmap to understand how we can accomplish the behavioral change we need to do. As the CEO of a national wellness based company, I see the daily struggles of patients trying to figure out how to feel better, often getting lost in their quest to understand the "how." I truly believe everyone will benefit by spending a few minutes a day using the resources of this Journal to reflect on their personal wellness goal(s). Change is often difficult. Make a personal commitment to living life to its fullest. Become aware of wellness. There is no greater gift you could give yourself!*

Jim Zechman, Chairman and CEO,
Alternative Medicine Integration Group, L.P.

I encourage my patients, my friends and my family to believe that they have the power within themselves to choose health as opposed to reacting to disease. Barbara Appelbaum's journal is a valuable tool that encourages and inspires each of us to achieve our wellness goals and create a balanced and healthy lifestyle. Your best you is within reach... Go For It!

Dino Mantis, DDS FICOI
Mantis Dentistry

As a neurosurgeon I recommend you have all your medical information available at a moment's notice. There is no universal repository for patient information. Therefore, it is your responsibility to have all your records organized, updated, and ready to share with your health care team, whether it is for a routine appointment or emergency care.

Having this on hand could save your life. This journal helps empower patients to be in control of their health instead of being a victim of it. It is a tool to help you achieve optimal health by visualizing your goals and facilitating preventative care.

> Clara Raquel Epstein, MD, FICS Neurosurgeon/CEO ENC/ENF
> The Epstein Neurosurgery Center, LLC
> The Epstein Neurosurgery Foundation, Inc. 501(c)(3)
> "Exceptional Neurosurgical Care"
> www.epsteincenter.com
> Twitter @TheNeurosurgeon

As a breast cancer survivor and coach I feel that Live in Wellness Now *is a valuable and useful resource on wellness. It is a great asset to anyone who is stuck in "sick" care on the journey to improved health. This journal offers practical and sensible approaches to enjoy our lives by empowering our own selves to take charge. If living well is your goal, then this journal, written by Barbara B. Appelbaum, is your ticket to comprehensive wellness of mind, body and spirit.*

> Cindy Giles, ACC, CPC,
> Life Coach and Cancer Survivor

Barbara Appelbaum's Journal is quite wonderful. It is an excellent guide to wellness. Ms. Appelbaum's acknowledgement of the universal energy that is with and within all of us, and her acknowledgement that healing prayer leads to cure is a giant step in our pro-active life, embracing wellness. I am especially pleased that Ms. Appelbaum embraces the importance of gratitude. She recognizes that gratitude brings wellness. In my spiritual practice, there is nothing more powerful than being thankful and expressing it daily. This journal is superb, a valuable tool for tracking our well-being. I will be sharing this journal with members of my spiritual community.

> Rabbi Dr. Douglas Goldhamer,
> Senior Rabbi, Congregation Bene Shalom, and
> President, Hebrew Seminary of the Deaf

The perfect addition to enhance anyone's health and wellness plan is Barbara Appelbaum's journal, **Live in Wellness Now.** *As someone who specializes in how to share more appreciation, I know that this is especially important to show to yourself. Establishing a quick yet powerful practice of giving yourself more compliments is one aspect of an empowered wellness action to fortify your spiritual and physical well-being, and part of what Barbara covers so well in this timely, important and especially helpful journal.*

Monica Strobel, Speaker, Trainer and Author of
*The Compliment Quotient: Boost Your Spirits,
Spark Your Relationships and Uplift the World*

Live in Wellness Now *is a "coach approach" to health that you will use for years to come. In a valuable journal form,* **Live in Wellness Now** *reveals the power to and process of achieving a great nutritional plan for you by creating a paradigm shift in the way you look at prevention and true health care.*

Deborah Van de Grift, CPC,
Certified Health Coach

I am proud to see graduates like Barbara B. Appelbaum furthering the mission of Integrative Nutrition by empowering others to take responsibility for their own health. By exploring your eating and lifestyle habits, you will begin to trust your body and find your path to wellness.

Joshua Rosenthal, Founder and Director
of the Institute for Integrative Nutrition

Barbara B. Appelbaum lives her wisdom. The words on these pages reflect the path that she has walked on her own journey. As someone who works daily connecting people to life enhancing vacations, this journal will be a wonderful companion on their journey to living lives of optimal well-being.

Lori Feiner Goldberg, Owner,
The Spa Connection

DEDICATION

I want to thank my parents. As cliché as it might sound, they are my best friends, my support system, my everything. They have been my greatest advocates, always cheering me on to continued success. Without their love and support, I'd be lost. This is the first of many books I hope to publish, and it is with great pride that I dedicate this initial endeavor to them. Mom and Dad – I love you more.

ACKNOWLEDGEMENTS

This journal was inspired by the greatest gift I ever received: multiple sclerosis. Being diagnosed with a chronic illness has taken me down a road that certainly would have been less traveled by me had life remained the same. I owe MS my gratitude for forcing me to wake up and see clearly for the first time who I want to be and how I want to live. MS gave me the power to come into my own, no longer doing as I was told but pursuing what I wanted. Having a chronic illness has also awakened me to the preciousness of life and the value of being my own advocate. I have become keenly aware of when I can control my life and when I have to be gentle with myself and acknowledge my healthiest self.

I want to also mention the coaching schools where I received my training: the Institute for Integrative Nutrition (IIN) and the Institute for Professional Excellence in Coaching (iPEC). Not only did their programs educate me, the staff became like family. Since completing the programs, both schools remain part of my life, offering ongoing support, education and genuine friendship.

Finally, I am truly blessed to have loving, supportive family and friends in my life. Several special friends have endorsed this endeavor of mine because they recognize its potential to help so many and want to do what they can to ensure that all who need it, read it and use it. My "tribe" is my foundation of being, and I'm very grateful to all who are in it.

Thank you.

Life is about making choices.

When you believe in your choices, you will grow.

When you grow by defining your intentions and health goals, you will achieve.

When you achieve your health goals, you will discover a new dimension of wellness.

Be Present | Be Purposeful | Be Well

Live in Wellness Now

A Proactive Guide to Living Well

Name: _____

TABLE OF CONTENTS

Dedication	VII
Acknowledgments	VIII
Introduction	12
How to Use This Journal	14
Medical	17
Personal information	22
Emergency contacts	23
Contact information – medical	24
Family history	27
Tests dates and results	28
Conversing with your physician	32
Calendars	37
Additional journaling pages	49
Nutritional	55
Contact information – nutritional	63
Food diary	64
Healthful eating list/grocery shopping guide	80
Progress chart – nutritional	81
Additional journaling pages	85

Fitness	91
Contact information – fitness	97
Personal thoughts regarding fitness	98
Progress chart – fitness	99
Exercise journal	104
Additional journaling pages	109
Spiritual	115
Contact information – spiritual	120
Progress chart – spiritual	121
Gratitude journal	125
Inspirational poem	132
Additional considerations	133
Additional journaling pages	135
Conclusion	141
Programs and services	144
About the author	145
About Appelbaum Wellness LLC	146
Final thought	147

INTRODUCTION

According to the National Wellness Institute, "*Wellness is an active process through which people become aware of, and make choices towards, a more successful existence.*" Wellness is the foundation of a successful life. And it is the coming together of the mind, body and spirit in personalized harmony for you.

This journal is meant to be used to help guide you on your path to wellness. There are sections for documenting your medical, nutritional, fitness and spiritual information. Use it as your "toolkit" for living healthfully – to hold you accountable to your goals and as a guideline for measuring improvement – so you can achieve success.

Remember to keep your goals SMART (according to Wikipedia, "SMART is a mnemonic to guide people when they set objectives"):

- Specific
- Measurable
- Attainable
- Relevant
- Time-bound

As you progress through this toolkit, you will notice a shift from managing your sick care to managing your health care. You will educate and equip yourself to function at your highest potential. Best of all, you will change from reacting to responding when it comes to your well-being.

All of the following pages can be copied to add to your journal and use for weeks and months to come. It might also be useful to stick a few plastic inserts to the inside back cover of your journal to hold discs so you can keep all of your prescriptions and x-ray or MRI CDs together in one place. If you feel creative, use the optional blank pages for additional journaling or even drawing as it pertains to your wellness journey. The journal is set up so you can use parts or the whole. It's up to you!

Most important, consult your physician before starting any new wellness program. Be sure to tell him/her what you are currently doing and what you plan to do. Be open and honest to ensure your well-being.

This journal is intended for informational purposes only and is not meant as a substitute for the advice provided by your physician or other healthcare professional. You should not use the information in this publication for diagnosing or treating a health problem or disease.

HOW TO USE THIS JOURNAL

From the time I was born, I was raised in a safe, loving environment with a strong sense of doing the right thing, being grateful and being a good person. Like everyone in my family, I became well educated (receiving a bachelor's degree and two master's degrees) and quite successful in the business arena. Over half of my career was spent in the non-profit healthcare sector. And then in 2006 I was diagnosed with multiple sclerosis (MS). It would change everything.

Before my diagnosis I was living on autopilot; living a pleasant but unfulfilling, stressful life. Finding out that I had MS – a chronic, often disabling disease that attacks the central nervous system – helped me discover my true passion of helping others learn to live a healthy and meaningful life. With a renewed "stop and smell the roses" perspective, I sought out a new career.

After discovering the profession of coaching, I knew instantly it was the way through which I could share myself and my passion with the world. My professional training was completed through the Institute for Professional Excellence in Coaching (iPEC) and the Institute for Integrative Nutrition (IIN). Both curriculums afforded me the education and support I needed to develop a growing practice focused on wellness and an integrative approach to nutrition.

I created this journal to help you be proactive in regard to your own wellness. I believe that we live in a "sick-care" society; being reactionary when it comes to our health. This leaves it up to you to manage your own care. Unfortunately no one shows you how to do this. Yet today is your lucky day! Through the use of this journal and sharing some personal insights, I'm going to teach you how to manage your healthcare.

Instead of taking a pill every time you get sick, consider how it would feel to not get sick in the first place. Okay, realistically I cannot promise you'll never get sick; however, I can promise that by taking proactive steps toward wellness, you will experience illness less often. Approach your life from the position of choosing to make the healthiest life choices possible instead of being like Scarlet O'Hara from *Gone with the Wind*, exclaiming, "I'll think about it tomorrow." Guess what? Tomorrow is today, and my question to you is, "What are you waiting for? Aren't you worth it?"

How often do you feel like you're on autopilot? Are you always tired and stressed beyond your limit? Do you struggle to balance the demands of work and family, feeling that if something doesn't change you're simply going to break? With the ongoing support and direction this guide provides, you will be able to set and maintain goals to support sustainable changes that will improve your overall health and wellness.

Look, I get it. You're probably thinking that what I preach is all well and good, but what makes this something you really can maintain? My diagnosis of multiple sclerosis woke me up to living the life I *wanted* versus the one I thought I *should*. So often I find people act based on others' expectations in lieu of their own desires and we "*should*" all over ourselves every day. I learned that what I was told was eating healthfully, really wasn't. I learned that what I was taught was enough exercise, no longer was. And with an overabundance of medical information being thrown at me in a very short amount of time, I realized I needed a way to organize everything so as to become my own advocate. As a result, I walk my own talk each and every day authentically and with passion. Yes, I stumble at times; I'm human. Yet I get right back up again and keep moving forward. Imagine how empowered I now feel.

As you start to pay attention to the medical, nutritional, fitness and spiritual components of your life, you will discover the powerful connection between the quality of these and the quality of your life. Like me, you will become empowered to listen to and trust your own body, explore and experiment with different ideas, and take responsibility for the choices that you make so as to create a life you truly love, enjoy and are enthusiastic about.

Most important, remember that real, permanent change occurs in baby steps. Focus on what you can do, not on what you cannot, or worse, what others do. Comparing yourself to others and trying to be "normal" are highly overrated, so please don't get stuck on that. Just be you! You are fabulous the way you are.

Through dealing with my own health-related challenges, I have come to recognize the importance of having one place to document medical, nutritional, physical and emotional aspects of your life. Documenting your life's journey helps alleviate the stress of trying to remember appointments, tests, medications, symptoms, thoughts and questions. This is a resource that will continually evolve and hopefully inspire you to *Be Present, Be Purposeful and Be Well.*

To Your Wellness!

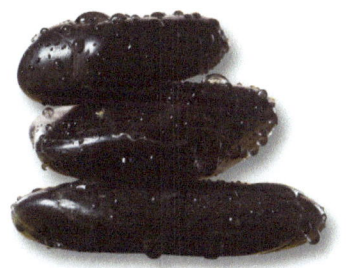

"Take care of your body with steadfast fidelity.
The soul must see through these eyes alone, and if they are dim,
the whole world is clouded."

Johann Wolfgang von Goethe

MEDICAL

Use this section to organize everything related to your medical needs. Keep a list of your emergency contacts and physicians, prepare for and track your medical appointments, maintain a list of your current medications and any pertinent tests, and chart your medical history along with that of your family. You will also find blank calendar pages to use for monthly reminders in regard to taking medications, scheduling appointments, etc., plus a notes section for documenting questions for your physician. By being prepared you will make better use of the limited time you have with your doctor.

Many of us fear going to the doctor. It's informally referred to as "White Coat Syndrome." You might notice this if your blood pressure mysteriously rises whenever you are in the doctor's office. So what can you do to alleviate your fear? After all, isn't the doctor supposed to be your friend?

Fear is not based on reality but on the expectation that what occurred in the past with negative results may happen again in the present or future. What if I told you that the feelings of fear are quite tangible? Fear can manifest as high blood pressure, anxiety/stress, a stomachache, muscle pain, or headache. In order to avoid real physical ailments like these, how can you empower yourself to be fearless?

Here are a few tips for overcoming fear when it comes to getting up the courage to visit your doctor:

1. Acknowledge your fear. It is simply an emotion that you're feeling because you are taking a risk, and that's a good thing. Trust your instinct to guide you appropriately.

2. Stop for a moment. Take a few deep breaths and calm down.

3. Focus your energy and thoughts to the present. Focusing on (or worrying about) past and future outcomes only fuels your fear.

4. Prepare for your doctor's appointment. Being proactive will help empower you to have a quality-packed appointment in which you can be open, honest and thorough with your physician.

Using these tips, you can decrease stress and result in a more productive meeting. Fear cannot have any power over you if you don't allow it to.

NOTES

Personal Information

Name: _____

Address: _____

Home Phone: _____

Work Phone: _____

Cell Phone: _____

Fax Number: _____

Email: _____

Specific Medical Information

Medications + vitamins (include dosages and frequency):

_____

_____

_____

_____

Allergies:

_____

_____

_____

Serious illnesses or recent hospitalizations (with dates):

_____

_____

_____

Emergency Contacts – Medical

Name: _____

Relationship: _____

Telephone: _____ Alt #: _____

Email: _____

Name: _____

Relationship: _____

Telephone: _____ Alt #: _____

Email: _____

Name: _____

Relationship: _____

Telephone: _____ Alt #: _____

Email: _____

Name: _____

Relationship: _____

Telephone: _____ Alt #: _____

Email: _____

Contact Information – Medical Physician

Physician Name: _____

Practice Name: _____

Address: _____

Telephone: _____

Cell: _____

Email: _____

Website: _____

Nurse's name(s): _____

Notes: _____

_____

Contact Information – Medical Other

Name: _____

Practice Name: _____

Address: _____

Telephone: _____

Cell: _____

Email: _____

Website: _____

Nurse's name(s): _____

Notes: _____

_____

Contact Information – Medical Other

Name: _____

Practice Name: _____

Address: _____

Telephone: _____

Cell: _____

Email: _____

Website: _____

Nurse's name(s): _____

Notes: _____

_____

_____

Contact Information – Dental

Dentist Name: _____

Practice Name: _____

Address: _____

Telephone: _____

Cell: _____

Email: _____

Website: _____

Nurse's name(s): _____

Notes: _____

_____

Family History – Medical

Father (living or deceased) – List any/all illnesses and age at diagnosis:

_____
_____
_____
_____
_____

Mother (living or deceased) – List any/all illnesses and age at diagnosis:

_____
_____
_____
_____
_____

Sibling (living or deceased) - List any/all illnesses and age at diagnosis:

_____
_____
_____
_____
_____

Sibling (living or deceased) - List any/all illnesses and age at diagnosis:

_____
_____
_____
_____
_____

Tests – Medical

Blood Test
Date: _____ Type of test: _____
Reason for test: _____
Results/Notes: _____

Blood Test
Date: _____ Type of test: _____
Reason for test: _____
Results/Notes: _____

Blood Test
Date: _____ Type of test: _____
Reason for test: _____
Results/Notes: _____

Blood Test
Date: _____ Type of test: _____
Reason for test: _____
Results/Notes: _____

X-Ray
Date: _____ Type of test: _____
Reason for x-ray: _____
Location taken: _____
Results/Notes: _____

X-Ray

Date: _____ Type of test: _____

Reason for x-ray: _____

Location taken: _____

Results/Notes: _____

Scan/MRI

Date: _____ Type of test: _____

Reason for scan/MRI: _____

Location taken: _____

Results/Notes: _____

Scan/MRI

Date: _____ Type of test: _____

Reason for scan/MRI: _____

Location taken: _____

Results/Notes: _____

For Women: Pap smear

Date: _____

Reason for pap: _____

Location taken: _____

Results/Notes: _____

For Women: Pap smear

Date: _____

Reason for pap: _____

Location taken: _____

Results/Notes: _____

Medical Live in Wellness Now

For Women: Mammogram

Date: _____

Reason for mammogram: _____

Location taken: _____

Results/Notes: _____

For Women: Mammogram

Date: _____

Reason for mammogram: _____

Location taken: _____

Results/Notes: _____

For Men: Prostate exam

Date: _____

Reason for exam: _____

Location taken: _____

Results/Notes: _____

For Men: Prostate exam

Date: _____

Reason for exam: _____

Location taken: _____

Results/Notes: _____

For both Men and Women: Dental exam

Date: _____ Procedure: _____

Reason for exam: _____

Results/Notes: _____

For both Men and Women: Vision exam

Date: _____ Procedure: _____

Reason for exam: _____

Results/Notes: _____

Conversation with Physician – Medical

Relationship status: _____

Children: _____

Pet(s): _____

Occupation: _____

Main health concerns:

_____

_____

_____

Any serious illnesses, hospitalizations or injuries?

_____

_____

_____

Number of hours of sleep you average per night: _____

Any pain, weakness, stiffness or swelling?

_____

_____

_____

What alternative therapies do you use (e.g. chiropractic, massage, etc.)?

_____

_____

_____

How often and what type of exercise you do?

_____

_____

Do you smoke or use drugs? If yes, how often and/or what type?
_____
_____

Other concerns you wish to share:
_____
_____
_____

Medical Live in Wellness Now

Write down any/all questions to ask your doctor:

Follow-up recommendations, tests, etc. (include dates and/or locations, if applicable):

Sometimes it's all too easy to forget when you are supposed to take your medicine and/or when certain symptoms manifested. Use the blank calendars on the next twelve pages – enough for an entire year – as a reminder tool to document your medication schedule, medical appointments, and other miscellaneous items such as workouts, illness onset, etc. Bring this with you to medical appointments, personal training sessions, meetings with your nutritionist and/or wellness coach, etc. as an aid for speaking with your practitioners. The more informed you and they are, the more productive your time together will be.

MONTH

Sun | Mon | Tue | Wed | Thu | Fri | Sat

Medical   Live in Wellness Now

MONTH _____

	Sun	Mon	Tue	Wed	Thu	Fri	Sat

Barbara B. Appelbaum

MONTH _____

Medical   Live in Wellness Now

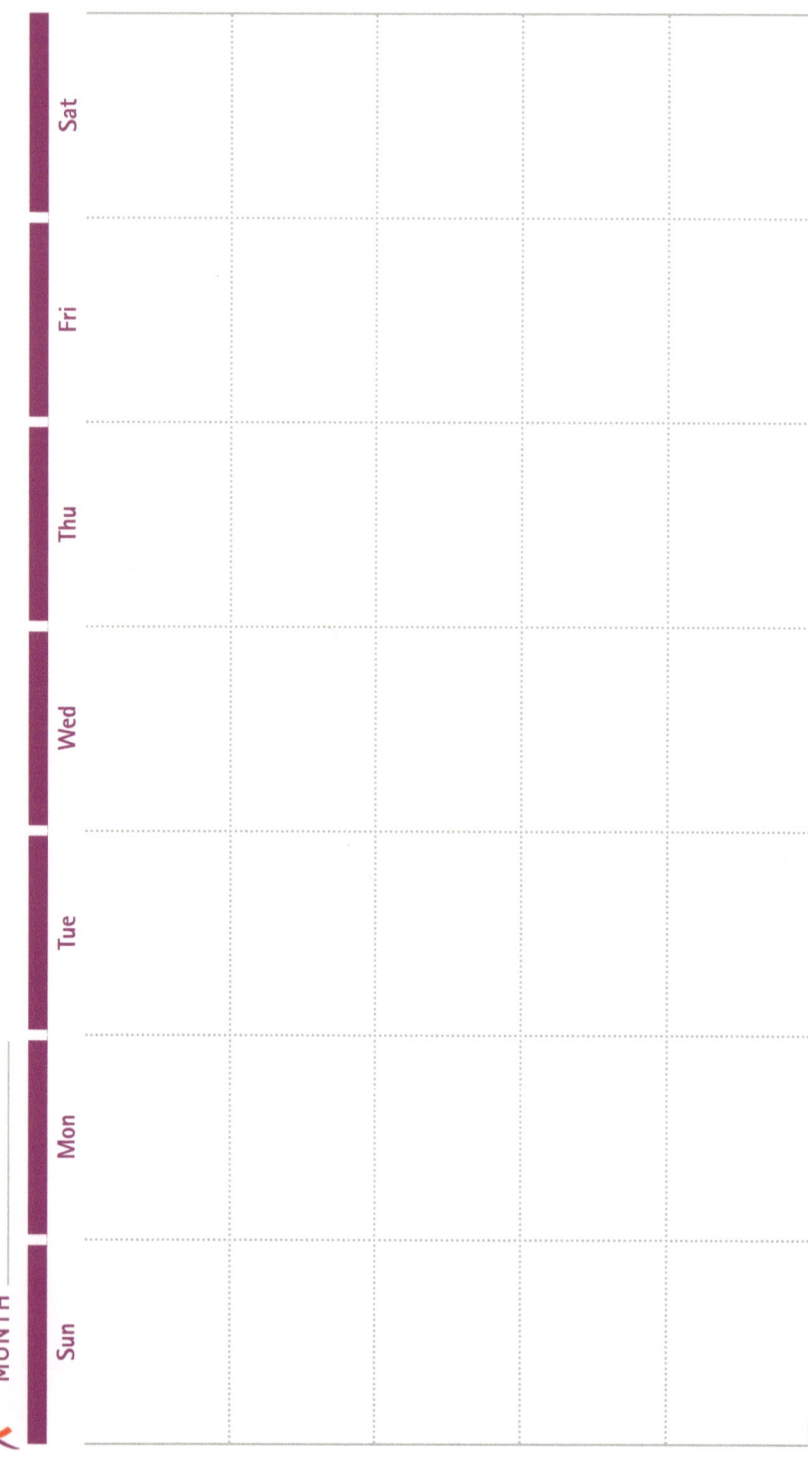

Barbara B. Appelbaum

MONTH _____

| Sun | Mon | Tue | Wed | Thu | Fri | Sat |

Medical

Live in Wellness Now

MONTH _____

Sun | Mon | Tue | Wed | Thu | Fri | Sat

Barbara B. Appelbaum

MONTH _____

Sun	Mon	Tue	Wed	Thu	Fri	Sat

Medical

Live in Wellness Now

MONTH _____

	Sun	Mon	Tue	Wed	Thu	Fri	Sat

Barbara B. Appelbaum

MONTH _____

| Sun | Mon | Tue | Wed | Thu | Fri | Sat |

Medical

Live in Wellness Now

MONTH _____

Sun | Mon | Tue | Wed | Thu | Fri | Sat

MONTH _____

Sun	Mon	Tue	Wed	Thu	Fri	Sat

Medical — Live in Wellness Now

MONTH _____

| Sun | Mon | Tue | Wed | Thu | Fri | Sat |

Barbara B. Appelbaum

ADDITIONAL JOURNALING PAGES

ADDITIONAL JOURNALING PAGES

ADDITIONAL JOURNALING PAGES

Medical — Live in Wellness Now

ADDITIONAL JOURNALING PAGES

ADDITIONAL JOURNALING PAGES

ADDITIONAL JOURNALING PAGES

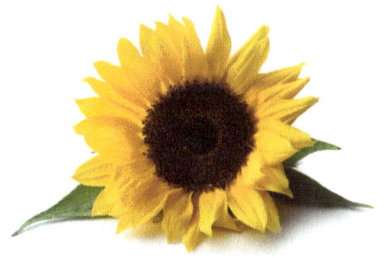

"Our food should be our medicine and our medicine should be our food."

Hippocrates

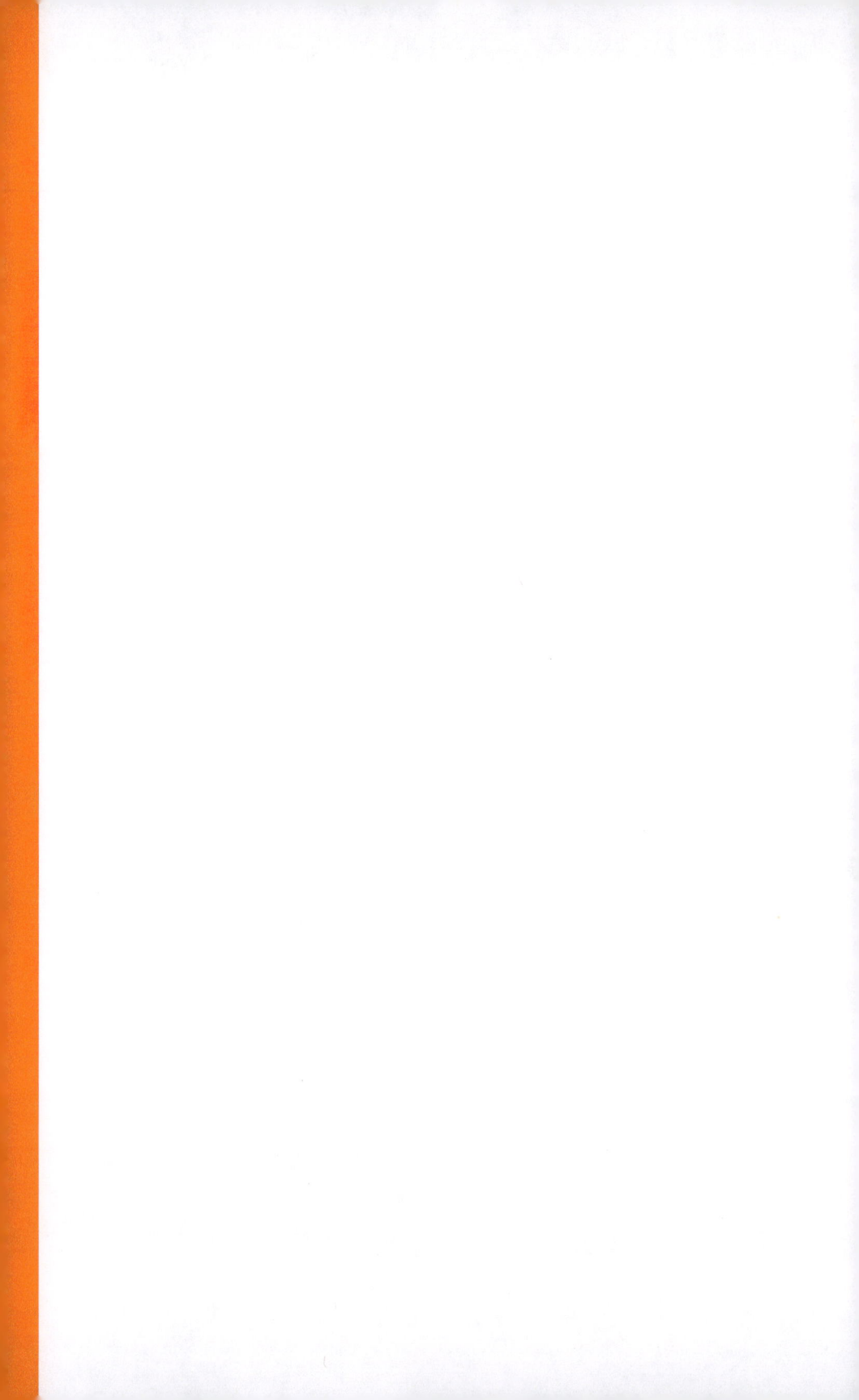

NUTRITIONAL

In my opinion, the key to effective healthcare is prevention. The use of food as medicine goes in conjunction with that. We truly are what we eat; it's that simple. I learned that it is best to eat *real* versus processed food. If you cannot pronounce the ingredients on the food label, you probably shouldn't be eating it. And the low-fat craze? Few nutrition and health experts think it's prudent to eat processed, low- or non-fat foods; they feel it is best to eat natural, whole-fat products in smaller quantities.

A great term I like to use is having a *food budget*. We have budgets for money, so why not have one for food? The term *diet* has earned a negative connotation, and the reality is that we ought to *eat right for life*. After all, food is nutrition that our bodies need.

Eating right for life is achievable if we create a budget for our eating. Namely, how much saturated fat will you allow yourself each day? How much protein? How much sugar and/or sodium? And so on.

If you have an issue with inflammation like I do, you'll want to keep your consumption of animal protein (meat, chicken, or fish) to a minimum. You can get the protein you need from other sources such as soy, nuts, or seeds. And when you choose to eat animal protein, select organic, hormone-free, and antibiotic-free when possible. Medical professionals maintain that sufficient protein is essential to good health particularly during stress or post-trauma (such as illness or surgery), because every cell in your body contains protein as its structure. It's part of your immune system, blood cells, etc.

Another essential element to your diet is a probiotic. Excellent probiotic sources are yogurt and oral supplements. They are particularly important to ingest when you are on antibiotics. Antibiotics kill bacteria but are unable to discriminate between good bacteria and bad bacteria. Probiotics replenish the good bacteria in your system which helps your immune system regain its strength.

Hydration is also a necessary consideration. Most Americans are dehydrated and hydrating your body is one of the easiest adjustments a person can make. Water composes 75% of your brain and muscles. It regulates your body temperature, helps your body absorb nutrients, aids in converting food to energy, eliminates waste, and more. How do you know if you're properly hydrated? It's simple. If your urine is light yellow or nearly clear, you are properly hydrated. If the color is dark yellow, go enjoy a glass or two of water and remember to do so regularly. Other drinks do not substitute for water. Try to get approximately eight 8 oz. glasses each day; more if you are exercising. Keep this in mind the next time you feel hungry. Sometimes hunger pains are mistaken for thirst. So grab a glass of water before you eat a full meal just in case you're actually thirsty and not hungry.

It is also important to note that it is best to toss out all artificial sweeteners. Yes, that includes all that diet soda you drink! You're much better off drinking water or tea and eliminating sugary drinks from your diet (and that includes fruit juice). Sugar drives hypertension; artificial sugar has proven to increase hunger, among other things. So if you must drink juice – I happen to love cranberry juice – get the 100% juice with no sugar added and dilute it with sparkling water and maybe add a lime. It's refreshing and healthy at the same time. By minimizing sugar, especially the artificial type, you will find foods that deliver a greater level of satisfaction and are healthier and more nutritious for your body.

In regard to cooking, it is best to cook foods at a moderate or low temperature to avoid chemical changes in the food. That is an important lesson if you are the king or queen of the BBQ and cook everything on "high" like I used to.

Whatever you choose to do with your eating habits, try to make choices that are healthy yet also fun and satisfying. That way the changes will be sustainable. And remember, lifestyle also plays a huge role in your eating habits. How you handle stress, how much exercise you get, and whether or not you practice meditation all play a role in your overall physical and emotional hunger. Keep in mind that the more you shift to healthier habits, the better you feel and the more you improve physically and mentally.

Use this section as a food diary to track your daily food and water intake. Notice your eating habits and changes in your mood related to eating, especially if you skip meals. Make note of anything you wish to discuss with your physician or wellness coach. There are fourteen (14) days' worth of spaces for entries. Copy these pages for tracking your food intake for at least one month to get a true understanding of what you are eating and to perhaps use as a conversation-starter with your doctor, nutritionist or health coach.

There are areas for recording what you eat, the amount, the caloric value, the number of grams of protein, and fat/fiber, if known (see Nutrition Facts label image). TOTAL up the number of each daily to see how much you are truly consuming. Use the Nutrition Facts labels on your foods to determine these numbers. Be careful when calculating! Make sure you are using the serving size indicated on the label and, for example, multiplying amounts by 2 if you eat double the serving size. Be sure to include everything you eat and drink (including water). Leave the space blank if the information is unknown. Use a reference book that lists food counts to assist you, if needed. The highlighted portions indicate the important facts to know about a food item before purchasing and/or consuming it:

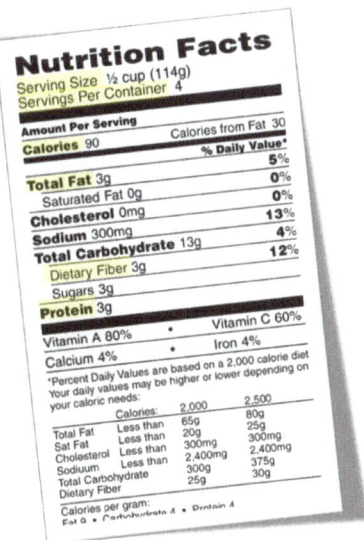

Food is what nourishes our bodies and provides a vital source of sustenance. And the body can only handle so much food intake.

Therefore it is imperative to fill it with healthy, nutrient-dense food so we garner the proper nutrition to healthfully thrive.

How often do you ask yourself, "Does this make me look fat?" Recently when getting dressed I came to a powerful realization as I silently asked myself for the umpteenth time in my life, "Does this outfit make me look fat?" For all of my adult life – and yes I mean all – I have not once looked in the mirror and thought I looked thin in whatever I was wearing. For as long as I can remember (maybe since the age of fifteen) I have felt fat even when I wasn't. Whether or not I was actually fat is not the issue. The true issue is that my self-image has always been skewed. Life has always been about eating too much, not eating enough, eating the wrong foods, eating the right foods, and so on. This obsession with food and weight isn't just a "girl" thing; everyone experiences it – male and female alike. Overall as a society we are obsessed with our physical image and equate it with feelings of success, or lack thereof.

Wherever you turn, photos are airbrushed, Hollywood stars are starving to be thin enough for the camera, diet commercials abound on television and many popular talk shows and self-help books focus on ways to become thinner. There are so many quick-fix fad diets out there it is overwhelming. "Drink this," "Cleanse that," "7 days to a perfect body," "Lose 10lbs in 3 days..." Wow, no wonder we tend to have poor self-images. All our lives we've been surrounded by messages that imply we are not good enough, and we grew up learning to take them to heart.

There is no cookie-cutter, one-size-fits-all solution or point of view. As an adult I'm learning to ignore those messages and follow what is healthy and right for my body. Of course I often think I'm not thin enough and wish my body looked differently; but then again, "thin enough" for what or whom? Why as a society are we so obsessed with weight equating to beauty and success? After all, that's really not true, and we'd all be much healthier if we embraced ourselves for who we are, not who or what we wish we could look like.

So how do you do this? Here are a few suggestions:

1. First and foremost, start with how you think. Focus on what you think is healthy for your unique body, mind and spirit, and what is achievable for you, not someone else.

2. Feel good about yourself. Create a daily mantra to remind you of all the positive characteristics you possess and the unique gifts you have to offer. Record it in this journal to look at again and again.

3. In striving to eat the best food possible as well as reduce unwanted cravings, try *crowding out* as an effective way to stop eating unhealthy foods. The idea of crowding out is that by adding more healthy foods to your diet you will crowd out the unhealthy foods. It is about giving yourself what you need; not denying yourself what you want. Take my one-week challenge: drink more water and eat nutritious, real food early in the day (hint: don't skip breakfast), and see if that doesn't crowd out your unhealthy cravings later in the day.

4. Most important, listen to your own body. It will tell you what it wants in order to live well. And be realistic. If weight loss is your goal, losing 1-2 lbs. per week is a sustainable rate that enables you to keep it off. If being healthy is your goal, try new nutrient-rich foods one at a time. Get used to them; learn how to cook with them; and then move on to another new item.

Remember to keep it real, keep it simple and keep it fun!

NOTES

Contact Information – Nutritional

Nutritionist or Health Coach's Name: _____

Practice Name: _____

Address: _____

Telephone: _____ Cell: _____

Email: _____

Website: _____

Notes: _____

_____

_____

Contact Information – Nutritional

Nutritionist or Health Coach's Name: _____

Practice Name: _____

Address: _____

Telephone: _____ Cell: _____

Email: _____

Website: _____

Notes: _____

_____

_____

FOOD DIARY EXAMPLE
Date: 2/11/13

	FOOD/AMOUNT	CALORIES	PROTEIN	FAT/FIBER
Breakfast:				
	Soy vanilla yogurt – 1	150	7	3/1
	Blueberries – ½ C	61	2	3/2
	Ground flax – 1 T	41	.5	4/3
	Coffee – 2 C			
Lunch:				
	Turkey sandwich:			
	W.W. Bread – 2 slices	200	8	3/8
	Mayo – 1T	90	0	10/0
	Lettuce + 1 slice tomato – minimal			
	Fresh Turkey – 4 oz.	193	3	5.6/0
	Strawberries – ½ C	23	.5	3/1.8
	Water – 16 oz.			
Snacks (optional):				
	Baby Bell Light mini cheese	50	6	3/0
	Medium apple	80	0	0/5
	Water – 16 oz.			
Dinner:				
	Stir Fry w/ Tofu:			
	Broccoli – 1C	44	5	.5/5
	Asian Mushrooms – 1C	80	2	.5/3
	Bok Choy – 1C	10	1	0/1
	Sprouted Tofu – 3 oz.	80	9	5/1
	Brown Rice – ½ C	150	4	1/2
	Olive Oil – 1T	120	0	14/0
	Lite Soy – 2T	20	2	0/0
	Water – 16 oz.			
	TOTALS:	**CALORIES**	**PROTEIN**	**FAT/FIBER**
		1,392	50	37.2/31.8

FOOD DIARY EXAMPLE
Date: 2/12/13

FOOD/AMOUNT	CALORIES	PROTEIN	FAT/FIBER
Breakfast:			
Eggs cooked in PAM – 2	150	12	10/0
W.W. Toast – 1 piece	100	4	1.5/4
Cantaloupe cubed – 1 C	56	1.4	.5/1.3
Raspberries – ½ C	31	.6	.3/4.2
Coffee – 2 C			
Lunch:			
Large Salad:			
Lettuce – 2 C	30	2	0/2
Tomatoes – ½ C	20	1	0/1
Sliced Colored Peppers – 1 C	25	.8	.2/1.7
Canned Tuna (water) – ½ can	60	13	.5/0
Olive Oil dressing – 2 T	120	1	13/0
Grated Parmesan – 2 T	20	2	1.5/0
Water – 16 oz.			
Snacks (optional):			
Almond Butter – 2T	180	5	16/4
Medium apple	80	0	0/5
Water – 16 oz.			
Dinner:			
Organic Salmon – 5 oz.	257	27	15/0
Asparagus (grilled) – 1 C	44	5	.6/4
Brown Rice – ½ C	150	4	1/2
Olive Oil – 1T	120	0	14/0
Small dinner salad:			
Lettuce – 1 C	15	1	0/1
Tomato	10	.5	0/.5
Italian dressing – 1T	60	.5	7/0
Water – 16 oz.			
TOTALS:	**CALORIES**	**PROTEIN**	**FAT/FIBER**
	1,528	80.8	68.1/30.7

Nutritional — Live in Wellness Now

FOOD DIARY
Date:

FOOD/AMOUNT   CALORIES   PROTEIN   FAT/FIBER

Breakfast:

Lunch:

Snacks (optional):

Dinner:

TOTALS: CALORIES   PROTEIN   FAT/FIBER

FOOD DIARY
Date:

                    FOOD/AMOUNT   CALORIES   PROTEIN   FAT/FIBER

Breakfast:

Lunch:

Snacks (optional):

Dinner:

                  TOTALS: CALORIES   PROTEIN   FAT/FIBER

Nutritional Live in Wellness Now

FOOD DIARY
Date:

                    FOOD/AMOUNT   CALORIES   PROTEIN   FAT/FIBER

Breakfast:

Lunch:

Snacks (optional):

Dinner:

                    TOTALS: CALORIES   PROTEIN   FAT/FIBER

Barbara B. Appelbaum

FOOD DIARY
Date:

FOOD/AMOUNT   CALORIES   PROTEIN   FAT/FIBER

Breakfast:

Lunch:

Snacks (optional):

Dinner:

TOTALS: CALORIES   PROTEIN   FAT/FIBER

Nutritional   Live in Wellness Now

FOOD DIARY
Date:

                    FOOD/AMOUNT   CALORIES   PROTEIN   FAT/FIBER

Breakfast:

Lunch:

Snacks (optional):

Dinner:

                    TOTALS: CALORIES   PROTEIN   FAT/FIBER

FOOD DIARY
Date:

FOOD/AMOUNT   CALORIES   PROTEIN   FAT/FIBER

Breakfast:

Lunch:

Snacks (optional):

Dinner:

TOTALS: CALORIES   PROTEIN   FAT/FIBER

Nutritional Live in Wellness Now

FOOD DIARY
Date:

                 FOOD/AMOUNT   CALORIES   PROTEIN   FAT/FIBER

Breakfast:

Lunch:

Snacks (optional):

Dinner:

                 TOTALS: CALORIES   PROTEIN   FAT/FIBER

FOOD DIARY
Date:

                      FOOD/AMOUNT   CALORIES   PROTEIN   FAT/FIBER

Breakfast:

Lunch:

Snacks (optional):

Dinner:

                      TOTALS: CALORIES   PROTEIN   FAT/FIBER

Nutritional   Live in Wellness Now

FOOD DIARY
Date:

                  FOOD/AMOUNT   CALORIES   PROTEIN   FAT/FIBER
Breakfast:

Lunch:

Snacks (optional):

Dinner:

                  TOTALS: CALORIES   PROTEIN   FAT/FIBER

FOOD DIARY
Date:

                    FOOD/AMOUNT   CALORIES   PROTEIN   FAT/FIBER

Breakfast:

Lunch:

Snacks (optional):

Dinner:

                    TOTALS: CALORIES   PROTEIN   FAT/FIBER

Nutritional Live in Wellness Now

FOOD DIARY
Date:

                    FOOD/AMOUNT   CALORIES   PROTEIN   FAT/FIBER

Breakfast:

Lunch:

Snacks (optional):

Dinner:

                    TOTALS: CALORIES   PROTEIN   FAT/FIBER

FOOD DIARY
Date:

                     FOOD/AMOUNT   CALORIES   PROTEIN   FAT/FIBER

Breakfast:

Lunch:

Snacks (optional):

Dinner:

                     TOTALS: CALORIES   PROTEIN   FAT/FIBER

Nutritional   Live in Wellness Now

FOOD DIARY
Date:

                     FOOD/AMOUNT   CALORIES   PROTEIN   FAT/FIBER

Breakfast:

Lunch:

Snacks (optional):

Dinner:

                     TOTALS: CALORIES   PROTEIN   FAT/FIBER

FOOD DIARY
Date:

                        FOOD/AMOUNT   CALORIES   PROTEIN   FAT/FIBER

Breakfast:

Lunch:

Snacks (optional):

Dinner:

                        TOTALS: CALORIES   PROTEIN   FAT/FIBER

Guidelines: Healthful Eating/Grocery Shopping

Vegetables* – approximately 5-6 servings/day
Dark, vibrantly colored throughout. A serving equals 2 cups, ½ cup chopped or cooked.

Fruit* – approximately 3-4 servings/day
Bold, deep colors; mixed berries are a great source of antioxidants. A serving equals ½ large fruit or 1 cup cubed/pieces.

Whole Grains and Starches – approximately 4 servings/day
High in fiber; starchy vegetables and beans included. A serving equals ½ cup cooked, 1 piece of bread, 1 small roll or muffin.

Lean Protein* – approximately 8oz/day
Choose lean proteins such as fish, beef, skinless chicken, cottage cheese (1/4 cup) or string cheese (1 ounce), eggs and egg whites (1 egg or 2 egg whites).

Healthy Fats* – approximately 4 servings/day
Limit hydrogenated and saturated fats from packaged foods and animal products. Choose vegetable fats such as olive oil when possible. A serving equals 1 teaspoon oil or 1 tablespoon salad dressing.

Dairy/Dairy Alternative* – approximately 2 servings/day
Low- or full-fat options and high in calcium; soy, almond, and rice milk included. A serving equals 1 cup milk or yogurt.

Nuts or Seeds – approximately 1 serving/day
Ground flaxseeds, chia seeds, walnuts, or pumpkin seeds high in omega-3 fats, or choose ½ an avocado to replace nuts. A serving equals ½ ounce or 2 tablespoons.

Bonus Treat (once in a while; not every day) – 1/day
A delicious example is 1-2 squares of dark chocolate > 70% cocoa, as a healthy treat.*

Use the above as a guideline; **find what works for you.** Every**body** is different.

*Choose organic when possible. Try not to consume diet foods that are processed. It is better to eat real, whole, and natural.

Use this form to chart your nutritional progress on a weekly or monthly basis. Notice how you feel physically and emotionally when you eat.

Date: _____

Today I feel: _____

My eating/nutritional goal is: _____

What will I do to achieve this? _____

What did I notice, if anything, by eating differently? _____

_____

Date: _____

Today I feel: _____

My eating/nutritional goal is: _____

What will I do to achieve this? _____

What did I notice, if anything, by eating differently? _____

_____

Date: _____

Today I feel: _____

My eating/nutritional goal is: _____

What will I do to achieve this? _____

What did I notice, if anything, by eating differently? _____

_____

Date: _____

Today I feel: _____

My eating/nutritional goal is: _____

What will I do to achieve this? _____

What did I notice, if anything, by eating differently? _____

_____

Nutritional   **Live in Wellness Now**

Date: _____

Today I feel: _____

My eating/nutritional goal is: _____

What will I do to achieve this? _____

What did I notice, if anything, by eating differently? _____

_____

Date: _____

Today I feel: _____

My eating/nutritional goal is: _____

What will I do to achieve this? _____

What did I notice, if anything, by eating differently? _____

_____

Date: _____

Today I feel: _____

My eating/nutritional goal is: _____

What will I do to achieve this? _____

What did I notice, if anything, by eating differently? _____

_____

Date: _____

Today I feel: _____

My eating/nutritional goal is: _____

What will I do to achieve this? _____

What did I notice, if anything, by eating differently? _____

_____

Date: _____

Today I feel: _____

My eating/nutritional goal is: _____

What will I do to achieve this? _____

What did I notice, if anything, by eating differently? _____

_____

Date: _____

Today I feel: _____

My eating/nutritional goal is: _____

What will I do to achieve this? _____

What did I notice, if anything, by eating differently? _____

_____

Date: _____

Today I feel: _____

My eating/nutritional goal is: _____

What will I do to achieve this? _____

What did I notice, if anything, by eating differently? _____

_____

Date: _____

Today I feel: _____

My eating/nutritional goal is: _____

What will I do to achieve this? _____

What did I notice, if anything, by eating differently? _____

_____

Nutritional Live in Wellness Now

Date: _____

Today I feel: _____

My eating/nutritional goal is: _____

What will I do to achieve this? _____

What did I notice, if anything, by eating differently? _____

_____

Date: _____

Today I feel: _____

My eating/nutritional goal is: _____

What will I do to achieve this? _____

What did I notice, if anything, by eating differently? _____

_____

ADDITIONAL JOURNALING PAGES

ADDITIONAL JOURNALING PAGES

ADDITIONAL JOURNALING PAGES

ADDITIONAL JOURNALING PAGES

ADDITIONAL JOURNALING PAGES

ADDITIONAL JOURNALING PAGES

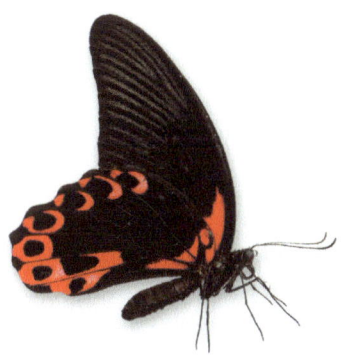

"We do not stop exercising because we grow old –
we grow old because we stop exercising."

Dr. Kenneth Cooper

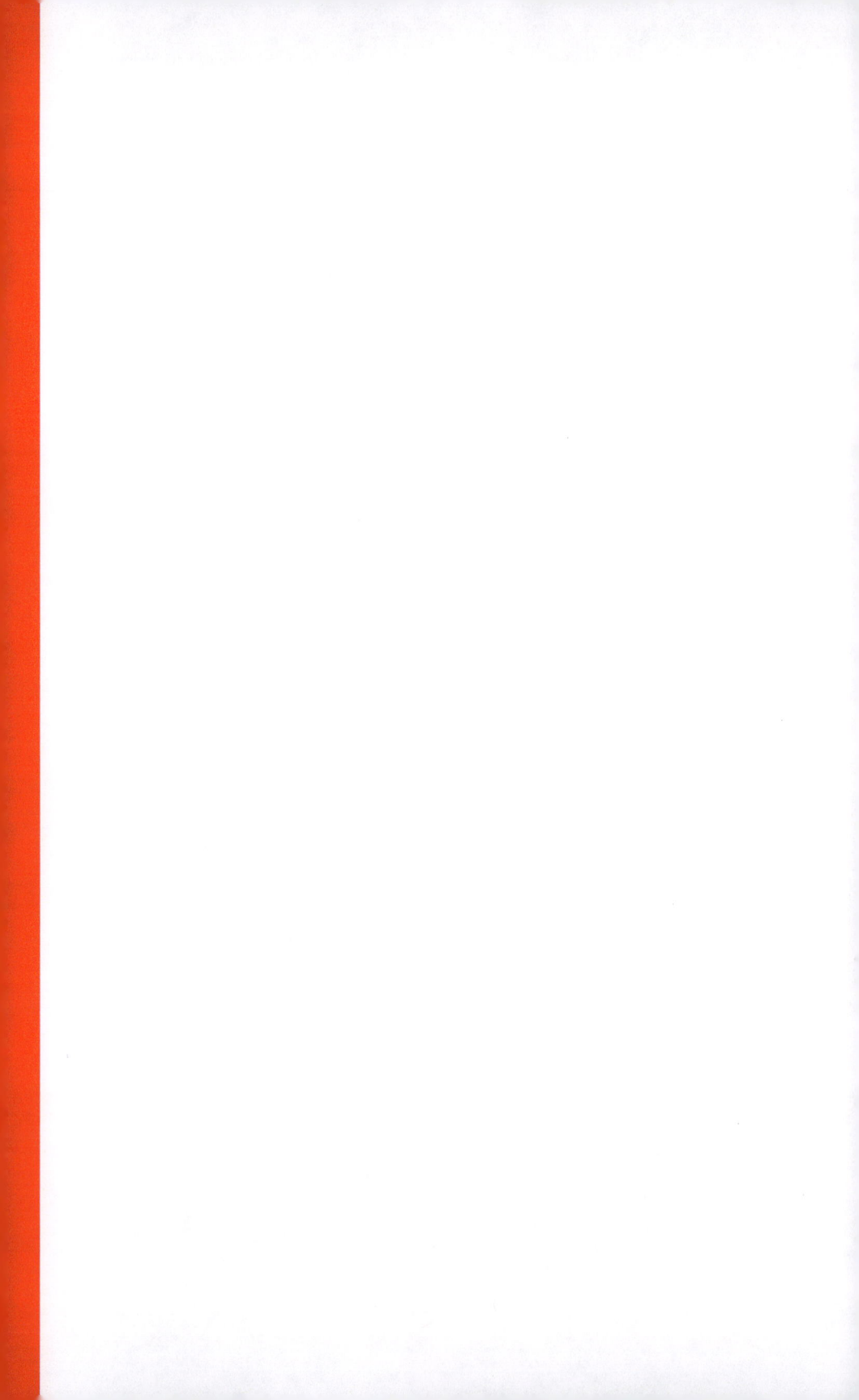

FITNESS

Exercise affects your physical and mental well-being for the positive. If you have never exercised before, start slowly and increase in small increments so as not to injure yourself. Keep in mind the old adage, "It takes 30 days to change a habit and 90 days to make it stick."

When you begin a new routine, start slowly, build up stamina and habit, and keep moving forward. Before you know it you'll notice a tremendous boost in your energy level and a more positive outlook. You will probably notice a decrease in stress, and you might even sleep better. When combined with a proper eating plan, you might also shed some of those unwanted pounds and/or build much needed muscle mass for strong bones.

Proper fitness is also essential for building energy and core stability. As you age, having a stable core will keep you physically well-balanced and help prevent falls, or at the very least minimize the damage you do to yourself during a fall. Exercise also prevents or minimizes joint pain.

Staying active is critical to staying healthy throughout life. With that said, it is okay to push yourself beyond what you think you are capable of, just not to the point of pain. Challenge yourself; don't be complacent. Exercise is one of the healthiest things you can do whether you are well or infirmed. Movement of any type is essential.

You may be asking yourself, "How do I fit this into my already busy day?" My answer to you is simple: This is your life. You only have one. So isn't it worth spending 30-60 minutes a day, 5-6 days per week focused on caring for you? If you don't focus on preventative care now, you will at some point in the future have to focus on reactionary care. Which would you prefer?

Here are some tips for starting an exercise program:

1. Put "*Me #1*" on your To-Do list. Schedule exercise on your calendar as if it is an important appointment you need to keep.
2. Pick an activity you enjoy that gets your heart rate up. Start by doing it a couple of times per week for 10-15 minutes and

gradually build up to 5-6 days per week for a minimum of 30 minutes. Some examples are walking, bicycling, swimming or even aerobics or zumba.

3. Add weight training to your routine twice per week. Enlist the assistance of a certified personal trainer or exercise physiologist to help you plan a customized routine for your specific capability and needs.

4. Team up with a friend, join a gym or go to group classes. It is always easier and more fun when you have someone with whom to share the activity.

5. Don't forget to leave time for stretching and/or deep breathing. Even practicing one of these for at least 10 minutes a day is beneficial. Keeping your body flexible is an integral component of good muscle health, and deep breathing is essential for supplying oxygen to all parts of the body.

6. Smile! When you smile it makes you (and others) feel happier and calmer.

7. Bonus: Exercise your brain to stave off age-related memory loss. Try puzzles, writing with your less dominate hand or even driving a new route to a routine destination.

Before being diagnosed with MS, my regular exercise routine was weight training twice per week, speed walking on flat terrain six days per week and perhaps a few rounds of golf during the summer months. I had to work at keeping my weight down (something I've had to do since saying goodbye to my twenties), yet was usually successful unless I completely let my eating get out of control. Throughout my thirties and early forties I belonged to a few health clubs, but never went on a regular basis. It took me years to realize how much I disliked the lighting and loud music in most clubs.

After MS, everything changed. Not only did my eating have to shift to an anti-inflammatory way of eating, but I had to learn how to exercise without heating up my core. Heat is the nemesis of MS in that it causes one's body to weaken. I also experienced a thirty-five pound weight gain from the medication I have to take. Upon enlisting the help of an exercise physiologist, I switched up my walking routine to that of interval training on the treadmill 5-6 days per week. I have kept up my weight training because I love it and it helps me stay strong. And I am now incorporating yoga, stretching and a bit of water exercise.

Now throw into the mix that I've started menopause and am over fifty. Life is a moving target and I keep myself active so as to keep up with it as healthfully as possible. Looking at me you would never guess I am over fifty or that I have MS. When people look at you, what do they see? No matter your limitations, likes or dislikes, find ways to keep moving and find what works for you.

NOTES

Contact Information – Fitness

Exercise Physiologist/Trainer Name: _____

Club/Gym/Practice Name: _____

Address: _____

Telephone: _____

Cell: _____

Email: _____

Website: _____

Member Number (if applicable): _____

Notes:

_____

_____

Contact Information – Fitness

Exercise Physiologist/Trainer Name: _____

Club/Gym/Practice Name: _____

Address: _____

Telephone: _____

Cell: _____

Email: _____

Website: _____

Member Number (if applicable): _____

Notes:

_____

_____

Personal Thoughts Regarding Fitness

What motivates me to exercise?
_____
_____
_____

What keeps me moving (e.g. music, books, a fitness partner, etc.)?
_____
_____
_____

Activities I like to do (list as much variety as possible):
_____
_____
_____
_____
_____
_____

How will I celebrate my success (possible rewards I will give myself)?
_____
_____
_____

Use the form to chart your progress on a weekly or monthly basis.

Date: _____

How am I doing today? _____

Exercise goal(s): _____

_____

How will I achieve this? _____

_____

How will I measure my success? _____

_____

Date: _____

How am I doing today? _____

Exercise goal(s): _____

_____

How will I achieve this? _____

_____

How will I measure my success? _____

_____

Date: _____

How am I doing today? _____

Exercise goal(s): _____

_____

How will I achieve this? _____

_____

How will I measure my success? _____

_____

Date: _____

How am I doing today? _____

Exercise goal(s): _____

_____

How will I achieve this? _____

_____

How will I measure my success? _____

_____

Date: _____

How am I doing today? _____

Exercise goal(s): _____

_____

How will I achieve this? _____

_____

How will I measure my success? _____

_____

Date: _____

How am I doing today? _____

Exercise goal(s): _____

_____

How will I achieve this? _____

_____

How will I measure my success? _____

_____

Date: _____
How am I doing today? _____
Exercise goal(s): _____
_____
How will I achieve this? _____
_____
How will I measure my success? _____
_____

Date: _____
How am I doing today? _____
Exercise goal(s): _____
_____
How will I achieve this? _____
_____
How will I measure my success? _____
_____

Date: _____
How am I doing today? _____
Exercise goal(s): _____
_____
How will I achieve this? _____
_____
How will I measure my success? _____
_____

Date: _____

How am I doing today? _____

Exercise goal(s): _____

_____

How will I achieve this? _____

_____

How will I measure my success? _____

_____

Date: _____

How am I doing today? _____

Exercise goal(s): _____

_____

How will I achieve this? _____

_____

How will I measure my success? _____

_____

Date: _____

How am I doing today? _____

Exercise goal(s): _____

_____

How will I achieve this? _____

_____

How will I measure my success? _____

_____

Date: _____

How am I doing today? _____

Exercise goal(s): _____

_____

How will I achieve this? _____

_____

How will I measure my success? _____

_____

Date: _____

How am I doing today? _____

Exercise goal(s): _____

_____

How will I achieve this? _____

_____

How will I measure my success? _____

_____

Exercise Journal

Use the following pages to log your daily physical activity. Copy the following pages as needed for additional space.

Gage the level of challenge by how out-of-breath you are. For example, Challenge level 1 is "no big deal," Challenge level 5 is "able to talk but breathing hard," while Challenge level 10 is "out of breath and can't talk." Better yet, invest in a Polar Heart Rate Monitor (or something similar) so you know exactly how hard you're working.

For health, try to exercise at least 30-60 minutes per day, 4-5 days per week. If weight loss is your goal, try to exercise 5-6 days per week and vary your routine to help the pounds melt away and keep it interesting and fun!

Don't forget the strength training! To build strong muscles and bones it is imperative to do this in addition to cardio. This is especially important for women to help stave off osteoporosis.

If you are totally new to doing a regular exercise routine, you might want to consult an exercise physiologist or certified personal trainer to get you started on the right path for you. Your body is unique and special, so give it the attention it deserves.

Set a goal to aim for and **always consult a physician before starting any new routine.**

Date: _____

Activity	Duration	Distance	Challenge level 0-10

Date: _____

Activity	Duration	Distance	Challenge level 0-10

Date: _____

Activity	Duration	Distance	Challenge level 0-10

Date: _____

Activity	Duration	Distance	Challenge level 0-10

Date: _____

Activity	Duration	Distance	Challenge level 0-10

Date: _____

Activity	Duration	Distance	Challenge level 0-10

Date: _____

Activity	Duration	Distance	Challenge level 0-10

WEEKLY TOTALS

Number of Times Exercised	
Average Duration	
Average Distance	
Average Challenge Level	

Date: _____

Activity	Duration	Distance	Challenge level 0-10

Date: _____

Activity	Duration	Distance	Challenge level 0-10

Date: _____

Activity	Duration	Distance	Challenge level 0-10

Date: _____

Activity	Duration	Distance	Challenge level 0-10

Fitness Live in Wellness Now

Date: _____

Activity	Duration	Distance	Challenge level 0-10

Date: _____

Activity	Duration	Distance	Challenge level 0-10

Date: _____

Activity	Duration	Distance	Challenge level 0-10

WEEKLY TOTALS

Number of Times Exercised	
Average Duration	
Average Distance	
Average Challenge Level	

Barbara B. Appelbaum

ADDITIONAL JOURNALING PAGES

ADDITIONAL JOURNALING PAGES

ADDITIONAL JOURNALING PAGES

ADDITIONAL JOURNALING PAGES

ADDITIONAL JOURNALING PAGES

ADDITIONAL JOURNALING PAGES

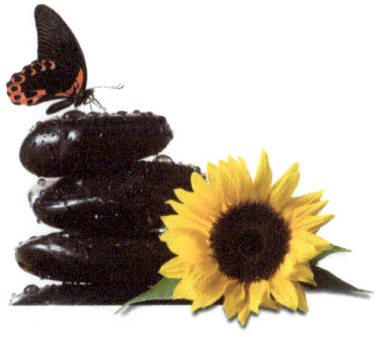

"When you change the way you look at things,
the things you look at change."

Dr. Wayne Dyer

SPIRITUAL

Energy is the universal life force. Some people refer to it as God or nature; others use different names. Through meditation and/or prayer, energy can be harnessed to heal the mind and body. It can also be appreciated through the expression of gratitude. Many ancient cultures practice energy rituals such as qigong, tai chi, yoga, meditation, healing prayer, etc. that have become popular in contemporary life due to their proven positive healing effects. When you practice any of these energy rituals, you allow your subconscious mind the ability to invite change so as to gain a greater sense of self and well-being.

Most problems and negative energy stem from your thinking. A regular spiritual practice helps you align with your inner core energy, shifting it to a higher level. It helps calm your mind and focus on your breath, quiets inner thoughts, reduces stress and allows your truth to unveil itself. A regular spiritual practice helps connect the body and mind for optimal wellness.

Meditation literally means "to think, contemplate, devise, ponder" according to Wikipedia. It is a mental practice used for the purpose of experiencing a heightened awareness within silence and relaxation. Scientists and physicians are researching the effects of meditation on the brain. For example, studies are showing that a regular practice of meditation provides these benefits:

- Improves mindfulness
- Promotes deep breathing
- Aids digestion
- Increases energy
- Reduces stress and frequency of illness
- Improves memory and brain health
- Improves overall wellness

There are many types of meditation, but the true essence is the same: it involves intention, focus and deliberate breathing. It also requires practice and dedication – change doesn't happen overnight.

For the past six years I have practiced healing prayer regularly, which most recently I have combined with yoga. I use the technique as a form of meditation that directs my thoughts inward energetically, helping me align my energy with that of the universe. Healing prayer is guided by the notion that one does not pray to be given strength; one prays to be cured. It uses principles for guiding our healing embraced by the Christian and Jewish traditions. Both faiths maintain that "When you pray, you pray as if your prayer has already been answered." And you pray with gratitude. As in yoga and other methodologies, when we direct our thoughts toward gratitude, our feelings and actions follow suit.

I'd like to share with you that MRIs of my brain show that my MS is progressing. Yet clinically speaking, my doctor says I am the healthiest patient he has. Therefore I ask you to use me as living proof that healing prayer and meditation work, and give it a try. It may not be a "cure" per say, but it does keep me healthy and I hope it does the same for you.

In the following pages you will find a section for keeping track of where and when you practice energy-type activities. There are also pages to copy so you can keep your own Gratitude Journal. A regular practice of gratitude helps you recognize and acknowledge a power (or energy) in the universe greater than you. With that energy working in tandem with your own, you become your best self. Keep in mind the adage, "Energy flows where attention goes."

Barbara B. Appelbaum

NOTES

Contact Information – Spiritual

Practitioner Name: _____

Club/Gym/Practice Name: _____

Address: _____

Telephone: _____ Cell: _____

Email: _____

Website: _____

Member Number (if applicable): _____

Notes:

_____

_____

Contact Information – Spiritual

Practitioner Name: _____

Club/Gym/Practice Name: _____

Address: _____

Telephone: _____ Cell: _____

Email: _____

Website: _____

Member Number (if applicable): _____

Notes:

_____

_____

Use this form to chart your progress:

Date: _____

Today I feel: _____

My spiritual goal is: _____

What ritual will I do to achieve this? _____

In what way do I feel differently after practicing this ritual? _____
_____

Date: _____

Today I feel: _____

My spiritual goal is: _____

What ritual will I do to achieve this? _____

In what way do I feel differently after practicing this ritual? _____
_____

Date: _____

Today I feel: _____

My spiritual goal is: _____

What ritual will I do to achieve this? _____

In what way do I feel differently after practicing this ritual? _____
_____

Date: _____

Today I feel: _____

My spiritual goal is: _____

What ritual will I do to achieve this? _____

In what way do I feel differently after practicing this ritual? _____
_____

Spiritual — Live in Wellness Now

Date: _____

Today I feel: _____

My spiritual goal is: _____

What ritual will I do to achieve this? _____

In what way do I feel differently after practicing this ritual? _____

_____

Date: _____

Today I feel: _____

My spiritual goal is: _____

What ritual will I do to achieve this? _____

In what way do I feel differently after practicing this ritual? _____

_____

Date: _____

Today I feel: _____

My spiritual goal is: _____

What ritual will I do to achieve this? _____

In what way do I feel differently after practicing this ritual? _____

_____

Date: _____

Today I feel: _____

My spiritual goal is: _____

What ritual will I do to achieve this? _____

In what way do I feel differently after practicing this ritual? _____

_____

Date: _____

Today I feel: _____

My spiritual goal is: _____

What ritual will I do to achieve this? _____

In what way do I feel differently after practicing this ritual? _____

_____

Date: _____

Today I feel: _____

My spiritual goal is: _____

What ritual will I do to achieve this? _____

In what way do I feel differently after practicing this ritual? _____

_____

Date: _____

Today I feel: _____

My spiritual goal is: _____

What ritual will I do to achieve this? _____

In what way do I feel differently after practicing this ritual? _____

_____

Date: _____

Today I feel: _____

My spiritual goal is: _____

What ritual will I do to achieve this? _____

In what way do I feel differently after practicing this ritual? _____

_____

Spiritual Live in Wellness Now

Date: _____
Today I feel: _____
My spiritual goal is: _____
What ritual will I do to achieve this? _____
In what way do I feel differently after practicing this ritual? _____
_____

Date: _____
Today I feel: _____
My spiritual goal is: _____
What ritual will I do to achieve this? _____
In what way do I feel differently after practicing this ritual? _____
_____

Gratitude Journal – Spiritual

Date: _____

Today I am grateful for:

1. _____
   _____

2. _____
   _____

3. _____
   _____

By acknowledging that for which I am thankful, I feel:

_____

_____

_____

Date: _____

Today I am grateful for:

1. _____
   _____

2. _____
   _____

3. _____
   _____

By acknowledging that for which I am thankful, I feel:

_____

_____

_____

Spiritual   Live in Wellness Now

Date: _____

Today I am grateful for:

1. _____
   _____

2. _____
   _____

3. _____
   _____

By acknowledging that for which I am thankful, I feel:

_____
_____
_____

Date: _____

Today I am grateful for:

1. _____
   _____

2. _____
   _____

3. _____
   _____

By acknowledging that for which I am thankful, I feel:

_____
_____
_____

Date: _____

Today I am grateful for:

1. _____
_____

2. _____
_____

3. _____
_____

By acknowledging that for which I am thankful, I feel:

_____

_____

_____

Date: _____

Today I am grateful for:

1. _____
_____

2. _____
_____

3. _____
_____

By acknowledging that for which I am thankful, I feel:

_____

_____

_____

Spiritual Live in Wellness Now

Date: _____

Today I am grateful for:

1. _____
_____

2. _____
_____

3. _____
_____

By acknowledging that for which I am thankful, I feel:

_____
_____
_____

Date: _____

Today I am grateful for:

1. _____
_____

2. _____
_____

3. _____
_____

By acknowledging that for which I am thankful, I feel:

_____
_____
_____

Date: _____

Today I am grateful for:

1. _____
   _____

2. _____
   _____

3. _____
   _____

By acknowledging that for which I am thankful, I feel:

_____

_____

_____

Date: _____

Today I am grateful for:

1. _____
   _____

2. _____
   _____

3. _____
   _____

By acknowledging that for which I am thankful, I feel:

_____

_____

_____

Spiritual Live in Wellness Now

Date: _____

Today I am grateful for:

1. _____

2. _____

3. _____

By acknowledging that for which I am thankful, I feel:

_____
_____
_____

Date: _____

Today I am grateful for:

1. _____

2. _____

3. _____

By acknowledging that for which I am thankful, I feel:

_____
_____
_____

Date: _____

Today I am grateful for:

1. _____
_____

2. _____
_____

3. _____
_____

By acknowledging that for which I am thankful, I feel:

_____
_____
_____

Date: _____

Today I am grateful for:

1. _____
_____

2. _____
_____

3. _____
_____

By acknowledging that for which I am thankful, I feel:

_____
_____
_____

Inspirational Poem to Quiet Your Inner Critic

I am Fear.

I am the menace that lurks in the paths of life, never visible to the eye but sharply felt in the heart (and mind).

I am the father of despair, the brother of procrastination, the enemy of progress, the tool of tyranny.

Born of ignorance and nursed on misguided thought, I have darkened more hopes, stifled more ambitions, shattered more ideals and prevented more accomplishments than history could record.

Like the changing chameleon, I assume many disguises. I masquerade as caution. I am sometimes known as doubt or worry. But whenever I'm called, I am still Fear, the obstacle of achievement.

I know no master but one; its name is "Understanding."

I have no power but what the human mind gives me, and I vanish completely when the light of Understanding reveals the facts as they really are, for I am really nothing.

   - Lou Tice

May you find Understanding *through a regular spiritual practice and quiet the negative self-talk while shifting your energy levels to a higher, more positive and healthful level.*

Additional Considerations

Have you ever thought about lifestyle as part of your overall health and well-being? In an integrative approach to wellness, there are four integral components to consider in addition to the food you eat:

1. Relationships – are they nurturing or do they cause you duress and/or leave you isolated?
2. Physical activity – your body needs to move. Do you exercise adequately for your health?
3. Career – are you passionate about what you do and find joy in your daily work or are you in a stressful, toxic environment?
4. Spirituality – most people do not have a regular spiritual practice. Studies show that such a practice promotes wellness. Do you have a regular spiritual practice?

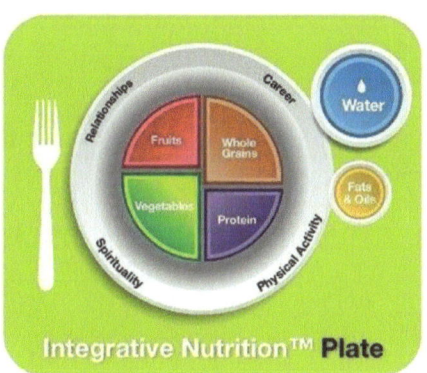

www.integrativenutrition.com

This is the Institute of Integrative Nutrition's version of our food plate. Notice the four words on the outer rim of the plate. These are the four lifestyle "foods" that should also be considered when you sit down to a healthy meal.

If you're curious as to whether your lifestyle is in balance, fill out my **Wellness Wheel of Life** (next page). Each of the eight sections represents a more detailed key component of your daily life.

Wellness Wheel of Life

For each section of the wheel, circle the number that represents your current level of satisfaction in that area of your overall wellness. The higher the number, the more satisfied you are in this area. Be honest.

When you connect the dots with a line, is a perfect circle created? Chances are the answer to that question is no. Where your line is not round represents disconnect in your life, causing you to experience a bumpy ride. Think of the wheel as a tire on your car. When it's flat, your ride is noisy, unstable and difficult to control. When the tire is properly inflated, your ride is quiet, smooth and controlled.

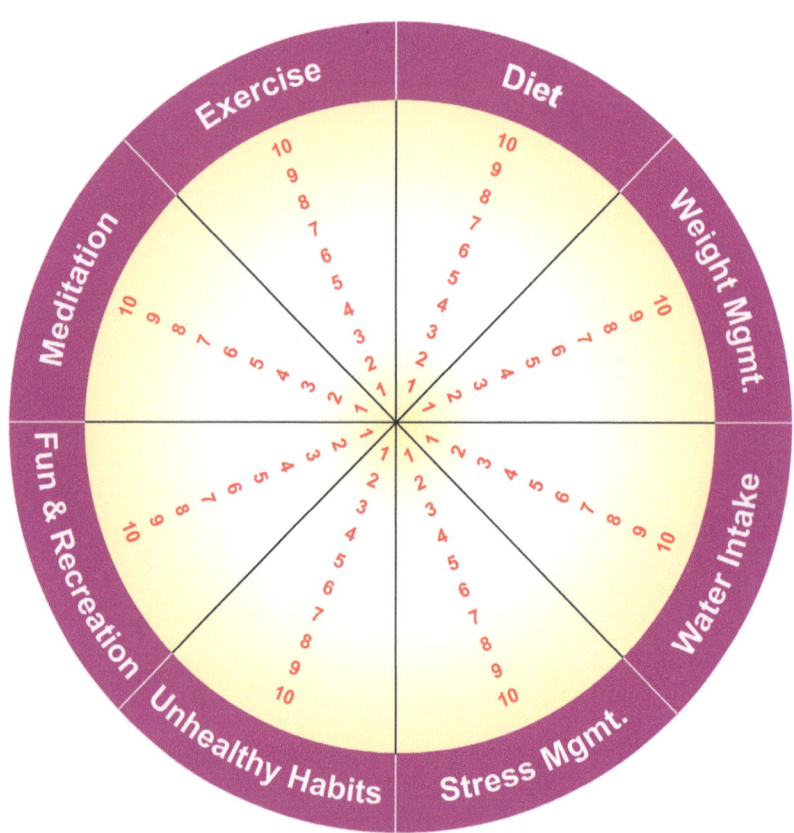

ADDITIONAL JOURNALING PAGES

ADDITIONAL JOURNALING PAGES

ADDITIONAL JOURNALING PAGES

ADDITIONAL JOURNALING PAGES

ADDITIONAL JOURNALING PAGES

ADDITIONAL JOURNALING PAGES

CONCLUSION

How many times in your life have you asked, "Why me?" How often have you felt like you just cannot get ahead, life is unkind, and no matter how hard you try, it still is not fair? You view life as a race to be won or lost, and filled with what one might call problems or challenges. Negative thinking can exacerbate the issue, turning whatever it is into a mountain instead of a molehill.

Every day can feel like an interminable challenge – the kids are out of control, your spouse depends on you for every little something necessary to get on with his/her day, the dog desperately needs walking, the phone doesn't stop ringing, at work your boss is yelling that he/she wanted the project completed yesterday, your co-workers look to you to take the blame if something goes wrong – and the list goes on and on. Just getting out of bed on some days can prove daunting. Is it any wonder we get through each day? Or isn't it?

If you take a moment in the middle of the chaos to just breathe, remember your inner strength and positive core energy, and focus on the opportunity instead of the challenge, how could life be different?

What if life were thought of as a marathon rather than a race? How would it feel to get off that proverbial hamster wheel and be in the moment? What would your life look like if you did not focus on stopping and starting, beginning and ending – but rather on living?

Hopefully this personal wellness journal will help you do just that. By tracking the medical, nutritional, fitness and spiritual aspects of your wellness, you will begin to focus on what's important in actually living your life. No longer will you live on autopilot. You will succeed in life because you have learned how to pay attention to all aspects of your mind-body-spirit connection. Use this tool to proactively achieve optimal wellness today and always.

If you want to learn more about taking control of your life, health and wellness, and need assistance along your journey, on the next page is a sampling of the programs and services offered by Appelbaum Wellness LLC for your consideration.

Be Present, Be Purposeful, Be Well

To Your Wellness!

PROGRAMS AND SERVICES

Appelbaum Wellness LLC offers individual coaching, group coaching, seminars, workshops, and keynote speaking. If you want personalized attention from a partner who will hold your agenda in confidence and without judgment, help you achieve results quickly, and hold you accountable when you stray off task, then look no further. We offer a diverse range of wellness solutions and products to fit the needs of any committed client. Below is a sample list of offerings. To learn more, visit our website now at www.appelbaumwellness.com.

It's Your L.I.F.E. – Live Inspired; Fully Engaged™ – Our signature program that teaches you to live in the moment and become an active participant in your life, health and wellness.

An Integrative Approach to Nutrition – This program will teach you how to have a holistic approach to your health and wellness. Simply stated, we will examine how all areas of your life are connected to what you eat and how they are affecting your overall health.

Health Wheel of Life – Are you having trouble determining whether or not your wellness is in balance? Learn how to use this tool as a visual aid for keeping your mind-body-spirit in harmony.

Put Together Your Own Team of Experts – Whether you're sick or healthy, do you find it overwhelming to manage your own care? Do you even know where to start? I'll teach you.

Learning to View Adversity as a GIFT™ – Are you currently faced with an adversity, whether physical or emotional? Learn how to benefit from a positive shift in perspective.

Vision Board Creation – Learn a powerful tool for creating your ideal future using the powers of visualization and intention.

ABOUT THE AUTHOR

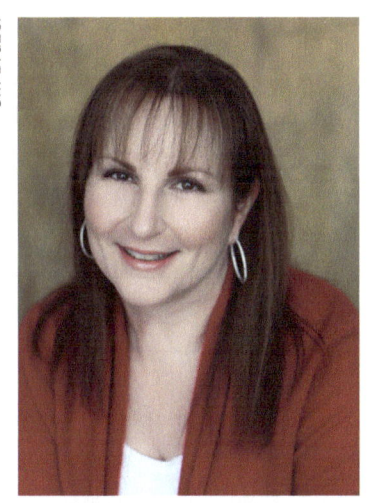

© Jill Brazel

Barbara B. Appelbaum, ACC, MBA, MAT, wellness coach, consultant, speaker, author, and founder of Appelbaum Wellness LLC has dedicated her life to assisting motivated Baby Boomers stave off age-related diseases as they grow older. She does this by helping them wake up to living their lives, seeing clearly what they want, and thereby achieving optimal wellness. She practices an integrative approach to health and wellness in which she explores how all areas of your life – mind, body, and spirit – are connected, and examines how they fit together and affect your overall well-being.

As a seasoned professional with over 26-years' experience, over half of which were in the healthcare sector, Barbara authentically walks-the-talk every day. After being diagnosed with multiple sclerosis in June 2006, her life changed forever. This "gift" made her realize the importance of waking up to actually living her life, learning the value of being her own advocate, and helping other people do the same.

Barbara is deeply committed to helping you learn to be proactive in your health care versus reactionary in your sick care, so you can feel great in your body and in your life. Her greatest wish is to never hear a person say, "I should be taking better care of myself."

Barbara is a certified member of the International Coach Federation (ICF), American Association of Drugless Practitioners (AADP) and an Ambassador for the National Multiple Sclerosis Society Greater Illinois Chapter.

ABOUT APPELBAUM WELLNESS LLC

COMPANY MISSION

Appelbaum Wellness LLC aims to create personalized best practices to teach people to be active participants in their life, health and wellness. We engage, motivate and inspire people to embrace a life of wellness so as to create the potential to be present, be purposeful and be well.

COMPANY VISION

Appelbaum Wellness LLC's vision is a tolerant world filled with like-minded, wellness-focused individuals who all choose to live healthfully and purposefully, and whose meaningful contributions impact themselves and society for the greater good.

For additional information about Appelbaum Wellness LLC, or to schedule Barbara for a presentation, please contact:
Appelbaum Wellness LLC
info@appelbaumwellness.com
Tel. 847-236-1330
www.appelbaumwellness.com

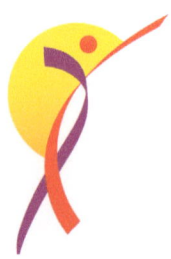

FINAL THOUGHT

The first wealth is health.

Emerson

Take care of your body. It's the only place you have to live.

Jim Rohn

What is your health worth to you?

www.ingramcontent.com/pod-product-compliance
Lightning Source LLC
Chambersburg PA
CBHW041616220426
43671CB00001B/4